TABLE OF CONTENTS

I0466832

INTRODUCTION

CHAPTER ONE

CHAPTER TWO

CHAPTER THREE

CHAPTER FOUR

2

INTRODUCTION

Skin cancer, a prevalent concern worldwide, has been the focus of significant research and awareness efforts due to its rising incidence and potential severity. As one of the most commonly diagnosed cancers, skin cancer encompasses a range of types, including basal-cell carcinoma, squamous-cell carcinoma, and melanoma. The impact of this disease extends beyond mere statistics, influencing countless lives with its implications for health and well-being.

In the quest to combat skin cancer effectively, dietary strategies have emerged as a crucial component in supporting overall skin health and potentially mitigating cancer risk. Research indicates that certain foods rich in antioxidants, vitamins, and healthy fats can play a pivotal role in strengthening the body's defenses against skin cancer. By integrating nutrient-dense foods into daily meals, individuals can enhance their skin's resilience, reduce inflammation, and support cellular repair processes.

This 7-day meal plan is meticulously designed to offer a balanced and varied diet tailored to bolster skin health and contribute to cancer prevention. Emphasizing a range of vibrant, whole foods, this plan incorporates a diverse array of fruits, vegetables, lean proteins, and healthy fats. Each meal is crafted to not only provide essential nutrients but also to deliver a rich and satisfying culinary experience.

By adhering to this meal plan, individuals can take proactive steps towards nurturing their skin and overall health. This plan serves as a practical guide for anyone looking to adopt a more health-conscious lifestyle, combining delicious, nutrient-packed dishes with the potential to support skin cancer prevention and overall well-being.

CHAPTER ONE

SKIN CANCER

Skin cancers are a group of cancers originating from the skin, characterized by the abnormal growth of cells with the potential to invade or spread to other parts of the body. They are the most frequently diagnosed type of cancer in humans. The primary types of skin cancer include basal-cell carcinoma (BCC), squamous-cell carcinoma (SCC), and melanoma.

Basal-cell carcinoma, which grows slowly, can cause local tissue damage but is less likely to metastasize or be fatal. It typically appears as a painless, raised area of skin, often shiny with small blood vessels visible on the surface, or as a raised area that may ulcerate. Squamous-cell carcinoma, on the other hand, has a higher tendency to spread. It usually manifests as a firm lump with a scaly top or may present as an ulcer.

Melanomas are the most aggressive type of skin cancer. They often appear as moles that change in size, shape, or color, have irregular borders, contain multiple colors, itch, or bleed. While basal-cell and squamous-cell carcinomas, along with other less common types, are collectively referred to as nonmelanoma skin cancers (NMSC), melanomas require more urgent and aggressive treatment due to their rapid progression and higher risk of metastasis.

Understanding the various presentations and characteristics of these skin cancers is crucial for early detection and effective treatment, emphasizing the importance of regular skin examinations and awareness of any changes in skin appearance.

Over 90% of skin cancer cases are attributed to ultraviolet (UV) radiation exposure from the sun. This risk is heightened across all three main types of skin cancer—basal-cell carcinoma, squamous-cell carcinoma, and melanoma. The increase in exposure is partly due to the depletion of the ozone layer, which allows more UV radiation to reach the Earth's surface. Tanning beds also represent a significant source of UV radiation, contributing to the incidence of these cancers. Notably, UV exposure during childhood is particularly detrimental for the development of melanomas and basal-cell carcinomas, whereas the risk of squamous-cell carcinoma is more closely linked to cumulative lifetime exposure to UV radiation.

Research indicates that between 20% and 30% of melanomas arise from pre-existing moles. Individuals with lighter skin tones are at a higher risk of developing skin cancer, as are those with compromised immune systems, whether due to medications or conditions such as HIV/AIDS. The definitive method for diagnosing skin cancer is through a biopsy, where a sample of the suspicious tissue is examined microscopically.

Preventive measures include reducing UV radiation exposure and consistently using sunscreen, which are effective strategies for lowering the risk of melanoma and squamous-cell carcinoma. However, the efficacy of sunscreen in preventing basal-cell carcinoma remains uncertain. Generally, nonmelanoma skin cancers are highly curable, primarily through surgical excision. In some cases, radiation therapy or topical medications like fluorouracil may be employed.

Melanoma treatment often involves a combination of surgery, chemotherapy, radiation therapy, and targeted therapy. For advanced cases where the cancer has metastasized, palliative care may be provided to enhance the patient's quality of life. Melanoma boasts relatively high survival rates, with over 86% of individuals in the UK and more than 90% in the United States surviving beyond five years after diagnosis.

Thus, public health efforts emphasize the importance of early detection and prevention to manage the risks associated with skin cancer effectively.

Skin cancer is the most prevalent form of cancer worldwide, comprising at least 40% of all cancer cases. The most frequently occurring type is nonmelanoma skin cancer, affecting an estimated 2 to 3 million individuals annually, although precise statistics are often lacking. Within the category of nonmelanoma skin cancers, approximately 80% are basal-cell carcinomas, and 20% are squamous-cell carcinomas. Despite their high incidence, basal-cell and squamous-cell carcinomas rarely lead to fatal outcomes, accounting for less than 0.1% of all cancer deaths in the United States.

Globally, melanoma, a more aggressive form of skin cancer, affected 232,000 people in 2012 and resulted in 55,000 deaths. The highest rates of melanoma are observed among white populations in Australia, New Zealand, and South Africa. Over the past two to four decades, the incidence of all three main types of skin cancer has significantly increased, particularly in regions with predominantly white populations.

This rise in skin cancer cases underscores the critical importance of preventive measures, early detection, and effective treatment strategies. The implementation of public health initiatives aimed at reducing ultraviolet radiation exposure, encouraging regular skin examinations, and promoting the use of sunscreen can play a vital role in managing and mitigating the global burden of skin cancer.

Furthermore, advancements in medical research and treatment

protocols continue to improve survival rates and quality of life for those diagnosed with skin cancer. The ongoing development of targeted therapies and comprehensive cancer care plans is essential to addressing the diverse challenges posed by this widespread disease. By fostering greater awareness and adopting proactive healthcare practices, the global community can work towards reducing the impact of skin cancer and enhancing patient outcomes.

CLASSIFICATIONS

Skin cancer is classified into three primary types: basal-cell carcinoma (BCC), squamous-cell carcinoma (SCC), and malignant melanoma.

Basal-cell carcinoma (BCC) is the most common form of skin cancer. It originates in the basal cells, which are located in the deepest layer of the epidermis. BCC typically manifests as a painless, raised area of skin that may be shiny with small blood vessels visible on the surface, or as a lesion that may ulcerate. Although BCC rarely spreads to other parts of the body, it can cause significant local damage if not treated promptly.

Squamous-cell carcinoma (SCC) arises from the squamous cells, which are found in the outermost layer of the skin. This type of skin cancer often appears as a firm, red nodule or a flat lesion with a scaly, crusted surface. Unlike BCC, SCC has a greater potential to spread to other parts of the body if left untreated, necessitating timely and effective intervention.

Malignant melanoma is the most serious and aggressive type of skin cancer. It develops in the melanocytes, the cells responsible for producing melanin, which gives skin its color. Melanoma can form in an existing mole that changes in appearance or as a new, unusual-looking growth. This type of skin cancer is known for its rapid progression and high risk of metastasis, making early detection and treatment critical for improving patient outcomes.

Understanding the distinct characteristics and behaviors of these three types of skin cancer is essential for effective diagnosis, treatment, and prevention. Medical professionals emphasize the importance of regular skin checks and protective measures against ultraviolet (UV) radiation to reduce the risk of developing skin cancer. Through education and proactive healthcare practices, individuals can significantly lower their chances of encountering these potentially life-threatening conditions.

Basal-cell carcinomas (BCCs) predominantly occur in areas of the skin that receive significant sun exposure, particularly the face. They have a low propensity to metastasize and rarely result in death. BCCs are typically treated effectively with surgical excision or radiation therapy.

Squamous-cell carcinomas (SCCs) are also common but are less prevalent than BCCs. SCCs have a higher likelihood of metastasizing compared to BCCs, although the overall metastasis rate remains relatively low. However, SCCs of the lip or ear, and those occurring in immunosuppressed individuals, exhibit a greater risk of spreading.

Melanomas are the least common of the three primary types of skin cancer but are the most aggressive. They frequently metastasize, and once they spread, they can be fatal.

In addition to these common types, there are several less frequent skin cancers, including dermatofibrosarcoma protuberans, Merkel cell carcinoma, Kaposi's sarcoma, keratoacanthoma, spindle cell tumors, sebaceous carcinomas, microcystic adnexal carcinoma, Paget's disease of the breast, atypical fibroxanthoma, leiomyosarcoma, angiosarcoma, and porocarcinoma.

Both BCC and SCC often exhibit a UV-signature mutation, indicative of UVB radiation-induced direct DNA damage as their primary cause. In contrast, malignant melanoma is predominantly caused by UVA radiation, which leads to indirect DNA damage through the generation of free radicals and reactive oxygen species.

Research has shown that the absorption of certain sunscreen ingredients into the skin, coupled with a 60-minute UV exposure, can increase the formation of free radicals if the sunscreen is applied in insufficient quantities and infrequently. However, modern sunscreens often exclude these specific compounds, and the combination of other ingredients tends to keep these compounds on the skin's surface. Additionally, frequent re-application of sunscreen can mitigate the risk of free radical formation.

The distinction between the types of skin cancer and their causes underscores the importance of protective measures against UV radiation, including the regular use of sunscreen, wearing protective clothing, and avoiding peak sun exposure times. Continuous advancements in sunscreen formulations and public health education are crucial in reducing the incidence and impact of skin cancer.

SIGNS AND SYMPTOMS

Skin cancer manifests through a wide array of symptoms, necessitating close attention to any unusual changes in the skin. Common indicators include persistent changes that do not heal, ulcerations, discoloration, and alterations in existing moles. For instance, a mole might develop jagged edges, increase in size, change in color, or exhibit a different texture. Additionally, a mole that begins to bleed is also a cause for concern.

Other prevalent signs of skin cancer include painful lesions that itch or burn, as well as large brownish spots with darker speckles. These symptoms can vary significantly depending on the type of skin cancer. For example, basal-cell carcinomas often present as shiny, translucent bumps, while squamous-cell carcinomas might appear as firm, red nodules or scaly, crusted lesions. Melanomas, on the other hand, are particularly noted for their ability to change an existing mole's appearance or form new, unusual growths with irregular borders and multiple colors.

Recognizing these symptoms early is crucial for effective treatment. Persistent monitoring of the skin and routine dermatological check-ups are essential strategies in the early detection of skin cancer. Public awareness campaigns and educational initiatives play a vital role in informing individuals about these symptoms, promoting proactive skin health practices, and encouraging timely medical consultation when suspicious changes are observed.

Moreover, advanced diagnostic techniques and treatment options have significantly improved outcomes for skin cancer patients. Innovations in medical imaging, biopsy procedures, and therapeutic interventions continue to enhance the precision of diagnosis and the efficacy of treatment, underscoring the importance of ongoing research and healthcare advancements in the fight against skin cancer.

Basal-Cell Skin Cancer

Basal-cell skin cancer (BCC) typically manifests as a raised, smooth, pearly bump on sun-exposed areas of the skin, such as the head, neck, torso, or shoulders. Often, small blood vessels, known as telangiectasia, are visible within the tumor. As the condition progresses, crusting and bleeding may develop in the center of the tumor, frequently causing it to be mistaken for a non-healing sore. BCC is considered the least lethal form of skin cancer and, with appropriate treatment, can be eradicated, usually without significant scarring.

Squamous-Cell Skin Cancer

Squamous-cell skin cancer (SCC) commonly appears as a red, scaling, thickened patch on sun-exposed skin. Some lesions present as firm, hard nodules and dome-shaped growths resembling keratoacanthomas. Ulceration and bleeding are potential developments in untreated cases, which may eventually grow into large masses. SCC is the second most common type of skin cancer and, while dangerous, it is not as perilous as melanoma.

Melanoma

Melanomas are typically characterized by a variety of colors, ranging from shades of brown to black. A minority of melanomas, known as amelanotic melanomas, appear pink, red, or flesh-colored and are often more aggressive. Warning signs of malignant melanoma include changes in the size, shape, color, or elevation of a mole. Additional symptoms include the emergence of a new mole in adulthood, pain, itching, ulceration, redness around the mole, or bleeding at the site. The "ABCDE" mnemonic is a helpful guide for identifying melanoma: A stands for "asymmetrical," B for "borders" (irregular, often described as "Coast of Maine sign"), C for "color" (variegated), D for "diameter" (larger than 6 mm, roughly the size of a pencil eraser), and E for "evolving."

Other Skin Cancers

Merkel cell carcinomas are usually rapidly growing, non-tender bumps that can be red, purple, or skin-colored. These tumors do not cause pain or itching and can be easily mistaken for cysts or other types of cancer. Due to their rapid growth and potential for metastasis, early detection and treatment are crucial.

Understanding the distinct presentations of various skin cancers is vital for early diagnosis and effective treatment. Regular skin examinations, awareness of changes in skin appearance, and prompt medical consultation are essential strategies in combating skin cancer. Public education and preventive measures, such as using sunscreen and avoiding excessive sun exposure, play a significant role in reducing the incidence of these cancers. Ongoing advancements in medical research continue to enhance diagnostic accuracy and treatment efficacy, offering hope for improved outcomes for individuals affected by skin cancer.

CHAPTER TWO

CAUSES

Ultraviolet (UV) radiation from sun exposure is the leading environmental cause of skin cancer, with significant risks for individuals in outdoor professions like farming. However, several additional risk factors also contribute to the development of skin cancer:

1. Light Skin Color: Individuals with lighter skin are more susceptible to skin cancer due to lower melanin levels, which provide less natural protection against UV radiation.

2. Age: The risk of developing skin cancer increases with age, as cumulative sun exposure over a lifetime can damage skin cells.

3. Smoking Tobacco: Smoking has been linked to a higher risk of squamous-cell carcinoma and other types of skin cancer.

4. Human Papillomavirus (HPV) Infections: HPV infections can

elevate the risk of developing squamous-cell skin cancer.

5. Genetic Syndromes: Certain genetic conditions, such as congenital melanocytic nevi syndrome, increase skin cancer risk. This syndrome is characterized by birthmarks or moles that appear at or shortly after birth, with larger nevi (greater than 20 mm) having a higher likelihood of becoming cancerous.

6. Chronic Non-Healing Wounds: Persistent wounds, known as Marjolin's ulcers, can evolve into

squamous-cell skin cancer if left untreated.

7. Ionizing Radiation: Exposure to ionizing radiation, such as X-rays, environmental carcinogens, and artificial UV radiation from tanning beds, significantly increases skin cancer risk. The World Health Organization has classified tanning bed users in the highest risk category for skin cancer, attributing hundreds of thousands of basal and squamous-cell skin cancer cases to these devices.

8. Alcohol Consumption: Excessive alcohol intake can increase the risk

of sunburns, subsequently raising the likelihood of developing skin cancer.

9. Immunosuppressive Medications: Use of immunosuppressive drugs, such as Cyclosporin A and azathioprine, significantly increases the risk of skin cancer. Cyclosporin A can raise the risk approximately 200-fold, while azathioprine increases it about 60-fold.

10. Alternative Wellness Behaviors: Practices like perineum sunning, where sensitive skin not typically exposed to sunlight is deliberately

exposed, can heighten the risk of skin cancer.

The combination of these factors underscores the importance of comprehensive skin cancer prevention strategies. These include minimizing UV exposure, using sunscreen, avoiding tanning beds, and being cautious with behaviors and substances that increase skin cancer risk. Additionally, regular skin examinations and prompt medical attention to suspicious changes in the skin are crucial for early detection and effective treatment. Public health initiatives and educational efforts play a vital role in raising awareness and encouraging protective measures against skin cancer.

Ultraviolet (UV) irradiation of skin cells results in DNA damage through specific photochemical reactions. One common form of this damage involves the formation of cyclobutane pyrimidine dimers (CPDs), where adjacent thymine or cytosine bases bond abnormally. These dimers are a frequent consequence of UV exposure and significantly disrupt the normal DNA structure, impeding essential cellular processes.

Human skin cells possess mechanisms to repair most UV-induced DNA damage through nucleotide excision repair (NER). This repair process identifies and excises damaged DNA segments, subsequently replacing them with the correct nucleotides, thereby safeguarding the skin against cancer development. However, the efficacy of nucleotide excision repair diminishes with excessive UV exposure. When the damage exceeds the repair capacity, unrepaired DNA lesions can accumulate, leading to mutations that may initiate the carcinogenic process.

The limitations of the skin's natural repair mechanisms under high UV exposure underscore the importance of preventive measures. Reducing direct sun exposure, wearing protective clothing, and consistently using broad-spectrum sunscreen are essential strategies for minimizing UV-induced DNA damage. Public health campaigns and educational programs play a crucial role in raising awareness about the risks of UV radiation and the importance of skin protection.

Moreover, ongoing research into enhancing DNA repair mechanisms and developing more effective protective agents continues to be pivotal in the fight against skin cancer. By understanding the molecular mechanisms of UV-induced DNA damage and repair, scientists aim to devise innovative approaches to bolster the skin's defenses and improve the outcomes for individuals at risk of skin cancer.

PATHOPHYSIOLOGY

Squamous-cell carcinoma (SCC) is a malignant epithelial tumor that primarily originates in the epidermis, squamous mucosa, or areas of squamous metaplasia. This form of cancer is characterized by its ability to invade and destroy the surrounding tissues.

Macroscopically, SCC often appears as an elevated, fungating mass, or it may present as an ulcerated lesion with irregular borders. Under microscopic examination, SCC tumor cells are seen to breach the basement membrane, forming sheets or compact masses that infiltrate the underlying connective tissue, known as the dermis. In well-differentiated carcinomas, the tumor cells are pleomorphic and atypical but still resemble normal keratinocytes from the prickle layer; they are large, polygonal, and have abundant eosinophilic (pink) cytoplasm with a central nucleus.

The organization of these tumor cells tends to mimic the normal epidermis, with immature or basal cells at the periphery gradually becoming more mature towards the center of the tumor masses. As these tumor cells undergo differentiation, they transform into keratinized squamous cells and form round nodules with concentric, laminated layers, known as "cell nests" or "epithelial/keratinous pearls." The surrounding stroma is typically reduced and contains an inflammatory infiltrate, primarily consisting of lymphocytes. Poorly differentiated squamous carcinomas, in contrast, contain more pleomorphic cells and lack keratinization, making them more aggressive and difficult to treat.

A significant molecular factor involved in the development of SCC is a mutation in the PTCH1 gene, which plays a crucial role in the Sonic Hedgehog signaling pathway. This mutation disrupts normal cellular signaling and contributes to the uncontrolled growth and invasion characteristic of SCC.

Understanding the pathological and molecular features of squamous-cell carcinoma is essential for accurate diagnosis and effective treatment. Advances in molecular biology and genetics continue to shed light on the mechanisms driving this cancer, paving the way for targeted therapies that improve patient outcomes. Public health initiatives focusing on prevention, early detection, and education about risk factors, such as UV exposure and smoking, are also vital components in the ongoing effort to reduce the incidence and impact of SCC.

CHAPTER THREE

DIAGNOSIS

The diagnosis of skin cancer typically involves a biopsy and histopathological examination, which are considered the gold standards for confirming the presence and type of skin cancer.

In addition to traditional diagnostic methods, several non-invasive techniques are employed to detect skin cancer. These methods include:

• Photography: Used for documenting and tracking changes in skin lesions over time.

• Dermatoscopy: Allows for the detailed examination of skin lesions, particularly helpful in diagnosing basal cell carcinoma (BCC) and aiding in skin inspection.

• Sonography (Ultrasound): Provides imaging of deeper skin structures and is used to assess the extent of skin lesions.

- Confocal Microscopy: Offers high-resolution imaging of skin layers and may assist in diagnosing certain skin cancers.

- Raman Spectroscopy: Analyzes molecular composition and can identify cancerous changes in skin tissue.

- Fluorescence Spectroscopy: Utilizes fluorescence to differentiate between normal and abnormal skin cells.

- Terahertz Spectroscopy: Investigates the properties of skin tissue at terahertz frequencies, which may reveal cancerous changes.

- Optical Coherence Tomography (OCT): Provides cross-sectional images of skin tissue. While OCT has shown potential in diagnosing basal cell carcinoma (BCC), its effectiveness for melanoma and squamous cell carcinoma (SCC) remains unclear and requires further research.

- Multispectral Imaging Technique: Captures images across multiple wavelengths to enhance the detection of skin abnormalities.

- Thermography: Measures skin temperature variations that may indicate the presence of cancer.

- Electrical Bio-impedance: Evaluates the electrical properties of skin to identify potential malignancies.

- Tape Stripping: Involves removing surface skin layers for analysis to detect abnormal cells.

- Computer-Aided Analysis (CAD): Systems that analyze images from dermatoscopes or spectroscopy to assist in detecting skin cancer. Although CAD systems are highly sensitive in detecting melanoma, they have a high false-positive rate. The current evidence is insufficient to recommend CAD over traditional diagnostic methods.

The utility of high-frequency ultrasound (HFUS) in diagnosing skin cancer remains uncertain, and there is limited evidence supporting the use of reflectance confocal microscopy for diagnosing basal cell carcinoma, squamous cell carcinoma, or other skin cancers.

The integration of these advanced diagnostic techniques, alongside conventional methods, aims to improve the accuracy and early detection of skin cancer. Ongoing research and advancements in technology continue to enhance the diagnostic capabilities and help refine the management of skin cancer.

PREVENTION

Sunscreen is widely recognized as an effective preventive measure against melanoma and squamous cell carcinoma, and its use is strongly recommended for reducing the risk of these types of skin cancer. However, evidence supporting the effectiveness of sunscreen in preventing basal cell carcinoma is limited. To further lower the risk of skin cancer, it is advisable to avoid sunburns, use protective clothing, wear sunglasses and hats, and minimize sun exposure, especially during peak sunlight hours. The U.S. Preventive Services Task Force advises individuals aged 9 to 25 to avoid ultraviolet (UV) light exposure as a precautionary measure.

Several strategies can help reduce the risk of developing skin cancer, including decreasing the use of indoor tanning devices and limiting exposure to the sun during peak hours. Increased application of sunscreen and the avoidance of tobacco products also play a significant role in lowering skin cancer risk.

Limiting sun exposure and avoiding tanning beds are critical because both involve UV light, which damages skin cells by inducing DNA mutations. These mutations can lead to the development of tumors and other skin growths. Besides UV exposure, other risk factors for skin cancer include having fair skin, a history of frequent sunburns, the presence of moles, and a family history of skin cancer.

Currently, there is insufficient evidence to support routine screening for skin cancers, and vitamin and antioxidant supplements have not demonstrated effectiveness in preventing skin cancer. While there is some tentative epidemiological evidence suggesting that dietary measures might reduce melanoma risk, this evidence lacks support from clinical trials.

For sun protection, sunscreens containing zinc oxide and titanium dioxide are commonly used to provide broad-spectrum protection against both UVA and UVB rays. These ingredients help shield the skin from the harmful effects of UV radiation.

Although consuming certain foods may help reduce the risk of sunburn, their protective effect is considerably less compared to the use of sunscreen. Consequently, sunscreen remains the most effective method for safeguarding the skin against the damaging effects of UV radiation and reducing the overall risk of skin cancer.

A comprehensive meta-analysis examining skin cancer prevention among high-risk individuals has identified significant findings related to topical and systemic treatments. The analysis revealed that the topical application of T4N5 liposome lotion effectively reduced the incidence of basal cell carcinomas in individuals suffering from xeroderma pigmentosum, a rare genetic condition that impairs the skin's ability to repair UV-induced DNA damage. Additionally, the study found that oral administration of acitretin, a medication often used to treat severe skin disorders, may offer protective benefits for individuals who have undergone kidney transplantation. This suggests that acitretin might help mitigate the increased skin cancer risk associated with immunosuppressive therapies used in transplant patients.

Furthermore, a study published in January 2022 reported promising advancements in skin cancer prevention through vaccination. This research highlighted a vaccine designed to stimulate the production of a specific protein essential to the skin's antioxidant defense system. By enhancing the skin's natural defenses against oxidative stress and DNA damage, this vaccine could potentially strengthen the body's ability to resist skin cancer development. This innovative approach represents a significant step forward in preventive oncology and underscores the ongoing efforts to improve skin cancer prevention strategies through novel therapeutic interventions.

CHAPTER FOUR

TREATMENT

The treatment approach for skin cancer varies based on several factors, including the type of cancer, its location, the patient's age, and whether the cancer is a primary tumor or a recurrence. For instance, in the case of a small basal-cell carcinoma in a young individual, treatments with high cure rates such as Mohs micrographic surgery or cryotherapy with topical chemotherapeutic agents (CCPDMA) may be recommended. Conversely, for an elderly and frail patient with multiple health complications, a basal-cell carcinoma located on a challenging area like the nose might be managed with radiation therapy, which, although having a slightly lower cure rate, might be preferable due to the patient's overall condition. In some cases, particularly for large superficial basal-cell carcinomas, topical chemotherapy might be chosen to achieve a favorable cosmetic outcome. However, this approach may not be sufficient for more invasive forms of basal-cell carcinoma or for invasive squamous-cell carcinoma.

Melanoma generally shows poor responsiveness to radiation and chemotherapy, making alternative treatments necessary. For low-risk skin cancers, options such as radiation therapy (either external beam radiotherapy or brachytherapy), topical chemotherapy (such as imiquimod or 5-fluorouracil), and cryotherapy (freezing the cancer) may provide effective control. However, these methods often have lower overall cure rates compared to certain surgical procedures. Other treatments for basal-cell carcinoma and squamous-cell carcinoma include photodynamic therapy, epidermal radioisotope therapy, electrodesiccation, and curettage, each of which offers different benefits and limitations.

Mohs micrographic surgery is a specialized technique used to excise cancerous tissue while preserving as much healthy surrounding tissue as possible. During this procedure, the removed tissue is immediately examined to ensure that no cancer cells remain at the margins, allowing for the precise removal of cancerous cells and optimal cosmetic results. This technique is particularly valuable for cancers in areas with limited excess skin, such as the face, and is known for its high cure rates comparable to those achieved with wide excision. Performing Mohs surgery requires specific training and expertise. An alternative technique, called CCPDMA, can be utilized by pathologists not trained in Mohs surgery and involves similar principles of removing cancerous tissue while minimizing impact on surrounding healthy tissue.

In cases where skin cancer has progressed and metastasized, additional treatments may be necessary, which could include more extensive surgical interventions or systemic chemotherapy.

For metastatic melanoma, a range of advanced therapies is available. These include biologic immunotherapy agents such as ipilimumab, pembrolizumab, nivolumab, and cemiplimab, which work by stimulating the immune system to target and destroy cancer cells. In addition, targeted therapies such as BRAF inhibitors—

vemurafenib and dabrafenib—and the MEK inhibitor trametinib are used to specifically target and inhibit cancer cell growth associated with genetic mutations in melanoma.

In February 2024, the U.S. Food and Drug Administration (FDA) approved a groundbreaking cancer treatment that utilizes tumor-infiltrating lymphocytes (TIL therapy). This innovative approach involves extracting and expanding a patient's own immune cells that are naturally capable of recognizing and attacking cancer cells. TIL therapy is now approved for use in melanoma cases that have not responded to other treatments.

Moreover, scientists are advancing the development of a personalized cancer vaccine, currently undergoing testing in an advanced clinical trial. This vaccine is designed to be tailored to the unique genetic characteristics of an individual's cancer, offering a potentially more precise and effective treatment option for those with resistant or recurrent melanoma.

Currently, surgical excision remains the most prevalent method for treating skin cancers. The primary aim of reconstructive surgery is to restore both the appearance and function of the affected area. The choice of reconstruction technique depends on factors such as the size and location of the skin defect. Reconstruction of facial skin cancers poses particular challenges due to the complex anatomy of the face, which includes highly visible and functionally critical structures.

For small skin defects, simple repair techniques are often employed. This involves approximating the edges of the skin and closing the wound with sutures, resulting in a linear scar. If the repair is aligned with natural skin folds or wrinkle lines, the resulting scar is less conspicuous. In contrast, larger defects may necessitate more complex repair methods, including skin grafts, local skin flaps, pedicled skin flaps, or microvascular free flaps. Among these options, skin grafts and local skin flaps are more commonly used.

Skin grafting involves covering a defect with skin taken from another part of the body. The graft is secured to the edges of the defect, and a bolster dressing is applied for seven to ten days to keep the graft in place while it heals. There are two main types of skin grafts: split-thickness and full-thickness. Split-thickness grafts are created by shaving a layer of skin from areas like the abdomen or thigh. The donor site heals within approximately two weeks. Full-thickness grafts, on the other hand, involve the complete removal of a skin segment, necessitating suturing of the donor site.

Split-thickness grafts are suitable for larger defects but may result in less aesthetically pleasing outcomes compared to full-thickness grafts, which are generally preferred for their superior cosmetic results.

However, full-thickness grafts are typically limited to small to moderate-sized defects due to their complexity.

Local skin flaps involve using tissue from the area surrounding the defect to cover the defect itself. This method allows for the use of skin that closely matches the defect in both color and texture. Various designs of local flaps can be employed to minimize damage to surrounding tissues and achieve optimal cosmetic results. Pedicled skin flaps involve transferring skin with its blood supply intact from a nearby body area. An example of this technique is the pedicled forehead flap, which can be used to repair large defects on the nose. Once the flap establishes a new blood supply from its new location, the original vascular connection can be severed.

PROGNOSIS

The mortality rates associated with basal-cell and squamous-cell carcinomas are relatively low, at approximately 0.3%, which translates to around 2,000 deaths annually in the United States. In contrast, melanoma, though less common, has a significantly higher mortality rate of 15–20%, resulting in about 6,500 deaths per year. Despite its lower prevalence, malignant melanoma accounts for approximately 75% of all skin cancer-related fatalities.

The prognosis for melanoma patients largely depends on the timing of treatment initiation. When melanoma is detected early, the chances of successful treatment are very high, particularly when the cancer can be surgically removed before it has spread. However, if melanoma has metastasized to other parts of the body, the outlook becomes considerably less favorable. As of 2003, Mohs micrographic surgery showed a high five-year cure rate of approximately

95% for recurrent basal-cell carcinoma.

In terms of skin cancer incidence, Australia and New Zealand report some of the highest rates globally, with nearly four times the incidence rates observed in the United States, the United Kingdom, and Canada. In these countries, around 434,000 individuals are treated annually for non-melanoma skin cancers, while approximately 10,300 individuals receive treatment for melanoma. Notably, melanoma is the most common type of cancer among individuals aged 15 to 44 in both Australia and New Zealand. The incidence of skin cancer in these regions has been on the rise. For example, in 1995, the incidence of melanoma among European descent residents in Auckland was 77.7 cases per 100,000 people per year. This rate was expected to increase in the 21st century due to factors such as local stratospheric ozone depletion and the delay between sun exposure and melanoma development.

A variety of skin tumors, both benign and malignant, can affect cats and dogs. In dogs, approximately 20–40% of primary skin tumors are malignant, while in cats, the rate is higher, ranging from 50–65%. While not all skin cancers in cats and dogs are linked to sun exposure, it can occasionally be a contributing factor. For dogs, areas such as the nose and the pads of the feet are particularly vulnerable as they lack protective fur and have more sensitive skin. Similarly, cats and dogs with thin or light-colored coats are at increased risk for sun-induced skin damage across their bodies.

As of 2010, skin cancers result in approximately 80,000 deaths annually, with 49,000 attributed to melanoma and 31,000 due to nonmelanoma skin cancers. This represents an increase from the 51,000 deaths recorded in 1990.

In the United States, over 3.5 million cases of skin cancer are diagnosed each year, making it the most prevalent form of cancer in the country. It is estimated that one in five Americans will develop skin cancer at some point in their lives. The most frequently diagnosed type of skin cancer is basal-cell carcinoma, followed by squamous-cell carcinoma. Unlike many other cancers, there is no dedicated national registry for basal-cell and squamous-cell skin cancers in the U.S.

In 2008, the United States reported 59,695 new cases of melanoma, with 8,623 deaths resulting from the disease. In Australia, more than 12,500 new melanoma cases are reported annually, with over 1,500 fatalities each year. Australia has the highest incidence rate of melanoma per capita in the world.

Despite a decline in the rates of many cancers in the U.S., melanoma incidence continues to rise. The National Cancer Institute reported approximately 68,729 new cases of melanoma in 2004.

In the United Kingdom, melanoma ranks as the fifth most common cancer, with around 13,300 diagnoses in 2011. It accounts for about 1% of all cancer-related deaths, with approximately 2,100 deaths in 2012.

Regarding non-melanoma skin cancers, which include basal-cell and squamous-cell carcinomas, about 2,000 deaths occur annually in the United States. This number has decreased in recent years. Most fatalities from non-melanoma skin cancers are among elderly individuals who may have delayed seeking medical attention until the cancer had advanced, as well as individuals with compromised immune systems.

MEAL PLAN

A meal plan for skin cancer focuses on incorporating a variety of nutrients known for their potential to support skin health, reduce inflammation, and potentially reduce the risk of cancer progression. Here's a 7-day meal plan that emphasizes antioxidant-rich foods, healthy fats, and lean proteins, while minimizing processed foods and excessive sugars.

Day 1

- Breakfast: Greek yogurt with mixed berries (blueberries, strawberries) and a sprinkle of chia seeds.

- Lunch: Grilled salmon with a side of quinoa and steamed broccoli.

- Snack: Carrot sticks with hummus.

- Dinner: Baked chicken breast with sweet potato mash and sautéed spinach.

- Dessert: Sliced apple with a handful of walnuts.

Day 2

- Breakfast: Oatmeal topped with sliced almonds, flaxseeds, and fresh blueberries.

- Lunch: Spinach salad with grilled chicken, cherry tomatoes, avocado, and a lemon-tahini dressing.

- Snack: A small handful of mixed nuts (almonds, walnuts, and cashews).

- Dinner: Turkey meatballs with whole grain pasta and a side of roasted Brussels sprouts.

- Dessert: A bowl of fresh strawberries.

Day 3

- Breakfast: Smoothie made with spinach, banana, almond milk, and a tablespoon of flaxseed.

- Lunch: Lentil soup with a side of mixed green salad dressed with olive oil and balsamic vinegar.

- Snack: Sliced bell peppers with guacamole.

- Dinner: Grilled tofu with a side of brown rice and steamed asparagus.

- Dessert: A small serving of mixed fruit (kiwi, pineapple, and mango).

Day 4

- Breakfast: Scrambled eggs with spinach and tomatoes, served with whole-grain toast.

- Lunch: Quinoa salad with black beans, corn, cherry tomatoes, and avocado, dressed with lime juice and cilantro.

- Snack: A handful of pumpkin seeds.

- Dinner: Baked cod with a side of roasted sweet potatoes and a mixed green salad.

- Dessert: Greek yogurt with a drizzle of honey and a few fresh raspberries.

Day 5

- Breakfast: Chia pudding made with almond milk and topped with fresh raspberries and a sprinkle of nuts.

- Lunch: Chicken and vegetable stir-fry with brown rice.

- Snack: A pear with a handful of sunflower seeds.

- Dinner: Stuffed bell peppers with lean ground turkey, brown rice, and vegetables.

- Dessert: A small bowl of baked apples with cinnamon.

Day 6

- Breakfast: Smoothie bowl with blended spinach, frozen berries, banana, and topped with granola and sliced almonds.

- Lunch: Mediterranean chickpea salad with cucumbers, tomatoes, olives, and feta cheese, dressed with olive oil and lemon.

- Snack: Sliced cucumber with a dollop of Greek yogurt dip.

- Dinner: Grilled shrimp with a side of farro and a mixed vegetable medley (zucchini, bell peppers, and onions).

- Dessert: A handful of fresh grapes.

Day 7

- Breakfast: Whole-grain avocado toast with a poached egg and a side of mixed fruit.

- Lunch: Butternut squash soup with a side of arugula salad with roasted beets and walnuts, dressed with a balsamic vinaigrette.

- Snack: Edamame pods with a sprinkle of sea salt.

- Dinner: Baked chicken thighs with a side of wild rice and roasted carrots.

- Dessert: A small bowl of fresh pomegranate seeds.

General Tips:

- Hydration: Drink plenty of water throughout the day.

- Portion Control: Adjust portions to meet your specific nutritional needs and energy requirements.

- Variety: Incorporate a variety of fruits and vegetables to maximize nutrient intake.

- Preparation: Opt for fresh, whole foods and avoid processed items as much as possible.

Always consult with a healthcare provider or a registered dietitian before making significant changes to your diet, especially if you have specific health conditions or dietary needs.

CONCLUSION

As we navigate the complexities of skin cancer prevention and management, it becomes increasingly clear that lifestyle choices, particularly dietary habits, play a vital role in supporting overall skin health. The 7-day meal plan presented is more than a collection of recipes; it represents a thoughtful approach to integrating nourishing, health-promoting foods into daily life. By focusing on foods rich in antioxidants, vitamins, and essential nutrients, this plan aims to fortify the body's defenses, reduce inflammation, and enhance the skin's ability to repair itself.

The path to better skin health is not solely about combating disease but also about embracing a holistic approach to well-being. Through careful selection of ingredients and mindful preparation, individuals can enjoy a diet that not only tantalizes the palate but also aligns with their health goals. This meal plan underscores the importance of preventive measures in the fight against skin cancer, offering a practical, actionable framework for those looking to make informed dietary choices.

Furthermore, adopting a lifestyle that prioritizes nutrient-rich foods contributes to a broader vision of health, where each meal serves as a building block for a resilient, vibrant life. It is essential to remember that while no single dietary change can guarantee immunity from skin cancer, consistent, healthy eating habits can significantly enhance overall wellness and potentially mitigate risk factors.

In conclusion, embracing this meal plan is a proactive step toward nurturing both skin and overall health. It reflects a commitment to not only enjoying a varied and delicious diet but also to making informed choices that align with long-term health objectives. As research continues to evolve, integrating such health-conscious strategies into daily life will remain a cornerstone of a comprehensive approach to preventing and managing skin cancer, ultimately contributing to a healthier and more vibrant future.

www.ingramcontent.com/pod-product-compliance
Lightning Source LLC
Chambersburg PA
CBHW071942210526
45479CB00002B/778